SELF CONTROL:

BEING IN CONTROL OF YOURSELF AND PERSISTING UNTIL YOU REACH YOUR GOALS

LARRY ASH

CONTENTS

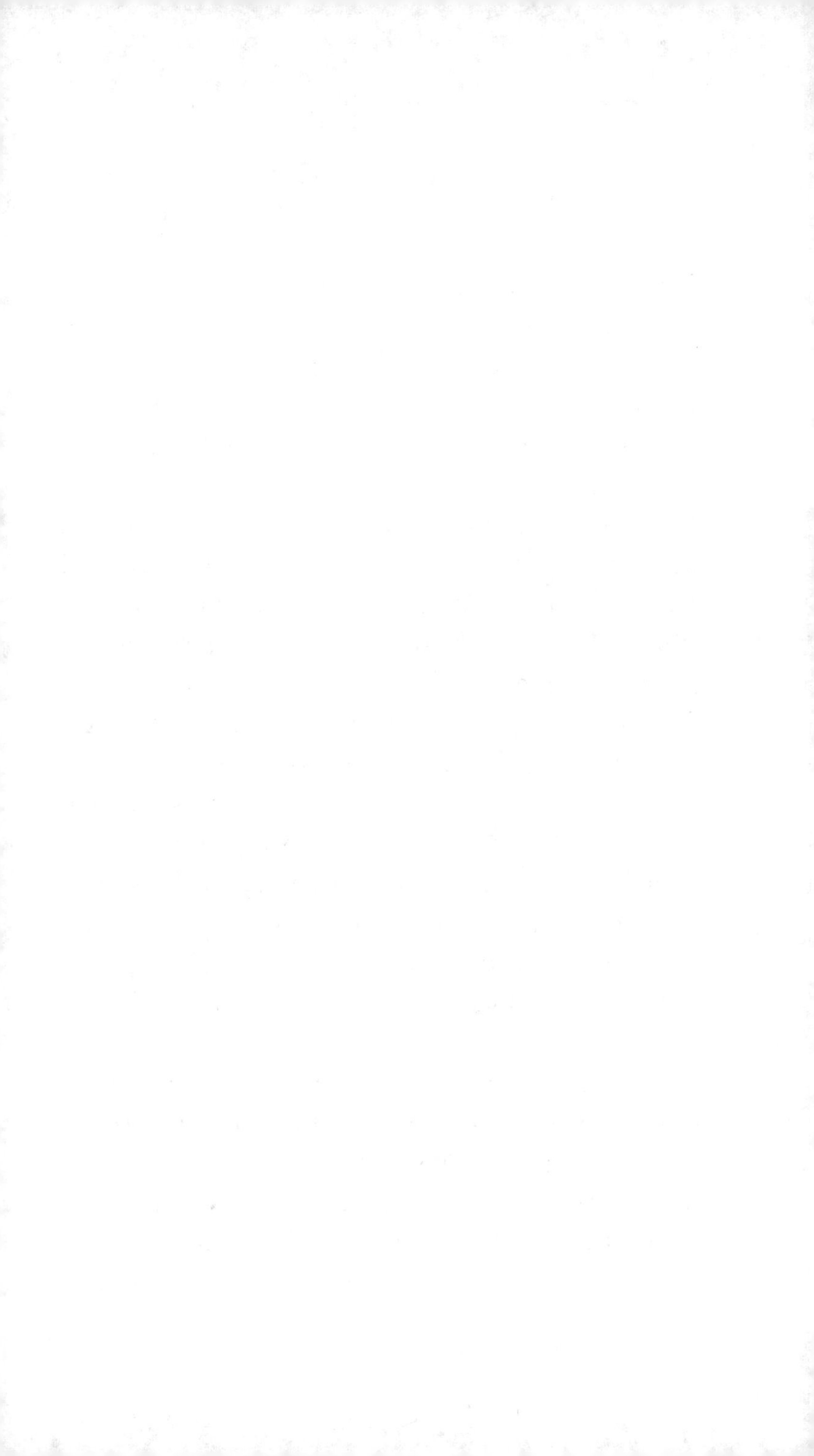

INTRODUCTION

Self-control is the ability to regulate and alter your responses in order to avoid undesirable behaviors, increase desirable ones, and achieve long-term goals. Research has shown that possessing self-control can be important for health and well-being.

 Self-control can be a difficult, lonesome process. But being disciplined will bring you practically endless benefits. Whatever you set your mind to, whether it be a short-term or long-term goal, is extremely likely to be accomplished if you have the discipline to put forth the effort required. Anything you desire to be is possible.

Knowing yourself can help you understand why you need self-control in your life and how to apply it. The next step is to imagine both your goals and the steps you must take to get there. You need a clear path to victory, so be as precise as you can and leave very little to chance.

One of the greatest equalizers known to man is self-control. You might begin at the bottom of your organization's hierarchy, but with perseverance and discipline, you'll eventually rise to the top. You may not have been lucky enough to have anything handed to you on a platter of silver, but with your determination and self-control, you'll soon surpass those who had a considerable head start.

If you apply all the strategies provided on this eBook, you'll be a self-control master in no time at all. With self-discipline, you'll have the mental strength to stop making excuses, you'll be able to resist any temptation that comes your way, and you'll find it easier to finally reach your goals in life.

KNOW YOURSELF

Self control

Let's start by deconstructing the term "self control" and defining its meaning. Self control is the capacity to exercise restraint or control over one's emotions, wants, and impulses. In other words, we have the ability to restrain ourselves from acting against our better judgment or experiencing negative emotions, especially when we are tempted. Self-control can also be referred to by other names including self-discipline, willpower, composure, and self-restraint.

Control is the ability to exert control over one's thoughts and behaviors in order to minimize unfavorable effects and enhance beneficial ones. The adjective self controlling, which is defined as "restraint of oneself or one's thoughts, feelings, responses, etc.

Know yourself

Knowing yourself is an important key to achieve self control. To learn your true self, identify your qualities, your fear, your strength, your weakness, your like and your dislike that make you unique. Daily reflection and meditation can help you cultivate a deeper understanding of your identity. As time goes on, you can build on these discoveries to create a deep and meaningful self control.

Ask yourself thoughtful questions. This knowledge can help you to know more about yourself. You can use this information to set some kind of goals to achieve your self control.

Some questions you can ask include:

- What do you love doing?
- What are your dreams in life?
- What do you want your legacy to be?
- What is your biggest criticism of yourself?
- What are some mistakes you've made?
- How do others perceive you? How would you like them to perceive you?

- Who is your role model? And so on.

Knowing your personality type will actually aid you in situations where you need self control and how to go about it.

FIND REASONS

Reason

Reasons are statements offered in explanation or justification for some belief, action, fact, event, etc.

In contrast to emotion, reason typically has to

do with thought and logic. People will think you are reasonable or have excellent reason, which indicates that you have thought things through. People will assume you have a valid cause for doing anything if they believe it to be so. Also when you reason, you consider all of the relevant factors before making a decision.

There must be reason why you need to control yourself.

For instance, you could find it tough to save money, and "to have savings" will be the reason why you need to have self control on the way you spend your mone, and this reason will motivate you to achieving your goals.

SET SMART GOALS

Setting goals is a well known approach to decision making with multiple criteria. You must develop SMART goals in order to have self-control and to make sure that your objectives are distinct and feasible.

Setting SMART goals means you can clarify your ideas, focus your efforts, use your time and resources productively, and increase your chances of achieving what you want in life.

SMART is an acronym that you can use to guide your goal setting, and SMART stand for:

- Specific (simple, sensible, significant).
- Measurable (meaningful, motivating).
- Achievable (agreed, attainable).
- Relevant (reasonable, realistic and resourced, results-based).
- Time bound (time-based, time limited, time/cost limited, timely, time-sensitive).

1. Specific

Your goal should be clear and specific, otherwise you won't be able to focus your efforts or feel truly motivated to achieve it. When drafting your goal, try to answer the five "W" questions:

- What do I want to accomplish?
- Why is this goal important?
- Who is involved?
- Where is it located?
- Which resources or limits are involved?

2. Measurable

It's important to have measurable goals, so that you can track your progress and stay motivated. Assessing progress helps you to stay focused, meet your deadlines, and feel the excitement of getting closer to achieving your goal. A measurable goal should address questions such as:

- How much?
- How many?
- How will I know when it is accomplished?

3. Achievable

Your goal also needs to be realistic and attainable to be successful. In other words, it should stretch your abilities but still remain possible. When you set an achievable goal, you may be able to identify previously overlooked opportunities or resources that can bring you closer to it.

An achievable goal will usually answer questions such as:

- How can I accomplish this goal?
- How realistic is the goal, based on other constraints, such as financial factors?
- How will it be possible

4. Relevant

This step is about ensuring that your goal

matters to you, and that it also aligns with other relevant goals. We all need support and assistance in achieving our goals, but it's important to retain control over them. So, make sure that your plans drive everyone forward, but that you're still responsible for achieving your own goal.

A relevant goal can answer "yes" to these questions:

- Does this seem worthwhile?
- Is this the right time?
- Does this match our other efforts/needs?
- Am I the right person to reach this goal?
- Is it applicable in the current socio-economic environment?

5. Time-bound

Every goal needs a target date, so that you have a deadline to focus on and something to work toward. This part of the SMART goal criteria helps to prevent everyday tasks from taking priority over your longer-term goals.

A time-bound goal will usually answer these questions:

- Whencan I do it
- What can I do today?
- Does my goal have a deadline?
- By when do you want to achieve your goal?

STRIKE THE BALANCE

Self-control is not about total abstinence, it's about finding the right balance to achieve the set goals.

It's been said that "a little of what you fancy does you good," and as long as it's not against the law or genuinely harmful, this proverb is almost probably accurate. Overindulging is bad, but denying yourself what you need is even worse. It will undoubtedly take a lot of joy out of your life quite quickly.

Thinking through your desires and imagining what "too little," "too much," and "just right" would look like will help you discover the correct balance.

Once you are aware, you may work toward finding the "just right" balance and are well on your way to learning self-control.

SET BOUNDARIES

You can pursue your goals with self control and avoid giving in to different temptations and distraction that will prevent you from reaching your objectives. Setting boundaries and developing the ability to say "no" when necessary will help you do this. Saying "yes" could be the courteous thing to do, but if it would hinder your achievement, you are better off saying "no."

You must be aware of your values, limitations,

likes and dislikes, and areas where you are willing to make concessions before you can set boundaries. While maintaining your boundaries, you must also be prepared to make concessions, especially if doing so will enable you to accomplish your objectives more quickly.

EMBRACE DISCOMFORT

At times, self-control can feel like hard emotional labor. In pursuing an ideal, you may need to let go of things that you like and accept some physical or emotional discomfort. Be prepared. Some sacrifice will almost always be required.

You only develop muscles by going through effort, sweat, and pain. You only write a great book by squeezing your mind and bleeding your soul through every sentence. You only develop inner strength by going through suffering with an open heart.

Discomfort is a form of pain, and our brain is programmed to avoid pain at all costs. By giving in to the brain, we shelter ourselves from pain, but also from life growth and from reaching out set goals. Our potential remains untapped.

SELF REWARD

As humans, we all love getting rewarded for our good deeds. And rewarding yourself is one of the most crucial components of self-control that we shouldn't ignore. We can accomplish our goals more quickly by reinforcing our established routines and behaviors with self-rewards.

If you don't regularly treat yourself, you'll discover that your motivation rapidly wanes and you may start putting on a mediocre show. You'll start to feel lethargic. While you could have completed the same task earlier in less than half the time, self control now would be a pain and a heavy burden.

However, not all awards are made equal. Avoid selecting a reward that may undermine your efforts to achieve your objectives. Keep in mind that you are awarding yourself for a job well done. Nothing you've done should be undone only to declare that you've given yourself a great reward.

The key takeaway here is that you have to choose a reward that's aligned with your goals. Never reward yourself with something that will undo your hard work, instead try to reward yourself with something that will help you reach your goals.

BUILDING GOOD HABIT

Developing good habits take time but since these are the main foundations for mastering self-control, I can assure you doing these is time well spent.

Habits are actions or behavior patterns that you do out of rote, out of repetition. It's become so ingrained in your daily life and you've become so used to it that you start doing it involuntarily. You don't even need to think about doing your habit before you do it, you just do. And in doing that, self control become so easy and become part of you.

Good vs Bad Habits

There are two types of habits. Good habits and bad habits. If you want to master self-control, you have to let go of your bad habits and replace them with new, positive ones.

Bad habits are negative behavior patterns that

are a hindrance or a roadblock to your mental and physical health, including any goals you' ve set for yourself. Laziness, unhealthy eating habits, rude behavior, bullying, swearing, and procrastination are examples of bad habits that really does nothing for you and does not contribute to your growth.

Of course, saying goodbye to a bad habit is easier said than done and is practically impossible to do overnight. It's called a habit because you do it involuntarily so it's going to take a lot of self- conscious effort on your part to stop doing your bad habits.

Some experts say it will take a minimum of 3 weeks to a month for a person to totally forego his bad habits. It will take plenty of mental and physical effort to do this but in the end, you'll be better off without your bad habits weighing you down.

So how do you replace a bad habit with a good habit?

Good habits come in many different forms. There are simple habits and there are physically demanding habits which might be difficult to master at first.

Assuming you're also working on breaking your bad habits, it would be best to start with a simple and easy-to-implement habit. After all, you don't want to overwhelm yourself and get stressed with the thought of doing too much at once. When overwhelmed, some people tend to procrastinate so working on too many habits at once may just backfire on you.

To narrow down some good habits you should pick up on, write down a list of habits you would like to acquire. If you really, really want to pick up an interesting but complicated habit, you can break it down into smaller bite-sized habits. Remember, it's easier to implement simple habits than highly complicated ones. Once you've written your proposed habits, write a score beside each habit and choose the one that came out easiest based on your scoring system.

Work on this habit every day for at least a month. Remember how in Chapter 2 we talked about journals and how you should be writing down everything you do in a day? Well, make sure this habit-forming activity of yours gets written down too. And don't forget to review your journal every week or so just to see how you're getting along with your progress.

When your new habit has finally become a real habit, it's time to work on the next positive habit you should acquire. Just rinse and repeat this process and try to retain as many positive habits as you can – habits that will help you fulfill your tasks at home, at work, or anywhere else.

Here's why building one good habit at a time is important for self-discipline success:

You're taking action. The more you take action, the more your new habit gets ingrained.

Your chances of failure are greatly reduced. Your good habits will be so ingrained in your brain that you do it by rote, without conscious thinking. If you committed the right action to memory, failing would be minimized.

It helps you build confidence and momentum. You're training yourself to be confident with one good habit. If you succeed, you'll feel pretty confident and you'd be encouraged to take on another positive habit.

It requires you to be responsible and accountable. Forming a good new habit will help you to become responsible since you've tasked yourself to do it repeatedly.

Here are a few examples of good habits:

Get up early in the morning (don't stay in bed until noon).

Exercise daily (even if you're busy, find a way to fit it into your schedule).

Eat a full breakfast (this is the first meal of the

day so don't skip it).

Drink plenty of water every day (stop drinking too many soft drinks).

Building good habits will help you master your self control.

CONCLUSION

Controlling yourself can be a long, lonely journey. But the rewards you'll reap with being disciplined is virtually limitless. Whatever you set your mind to do and achieve, whether it's a short term or long term goal, is very much possible if you have the self control to do what's necessary to achieve your goal. You can be anything you want to be.

Start off your journey by knowing your why and why you need self-discipline in your life. Then you need to visualize your goals as well as the processes you need to carry out to reach your goal. You have to have a roadmap to success so you need to be as specific as possible and leave very little to chance.

Striking your balance between your goals to help you achieve your goals is necessary.

To succeed at controlling yourself, you'll need to learn how to set boundaries and say no to temptations and distractions. You'll also need to stop sabotaging yourself and learn how to overcome your fears and insecurities because if you don't then you'll never leave your comfort zone and you'll never get anywhere in life.

Have self control is not an easy task, do there must be an ability to endure discomfort

Rewarding yourself also plays an important role in disciplining yourself especially if you apply delayed gratification. You can keep your mind focused on getting a reward for a job well done and you'll do your best to make sure you get that reward. And also Building a good, habit-forming routine that will help you achieve your goals is necessary.

Self-discipline is one of the greatest equalizers known to man. You may start off at the bottom rung of your organization but with hard work and discipline, you'll make it to the top, sooner or later. You may not have been lucky enough to have anything handed to you on a silver platter, but with your determination and self-self control, you'll soon surpass those who had a considerable head start.

If you apply all the strategies written on this Book, you'll be a self-discipline master in no time at all. With self-control you'll have the mental strength to stop making excuses, you'll be able to resist any temptation that comes your way, and you'll find it easier to finally reach your goals in life.

www.ingramcontent.com/pod-product-compliance
Lightning Source LLC
Chambersburg PA
CBHW071506150726
48000CB00006B/2715